LEADERSHIP FOR WELLBEING IN SCHOOLS

Dr. Abimbola Banu-Ogundere

Leadership for Wellbeing in Schools

CONTENTS

WHAT IS WELLBEING?

Wellbeing is a subjective term.

Wellbeing expresses a positive emotional state which is because of harmony between the sum of specific environment factors on one hand and the personal needs and expectations of the workforce on the other – Atterman at al, 2007.

Wellbeing means different things to different people: **quality of life or symptom of work life balance. To some a measure of stress is desirable to be high performing.**

Wellbeing can be personal where a personal is satisfied with life and is functioning positively with positive feelings. Wellbeing can be social, relating to positive supportive relationships, trust and belonging.

- Specific Environment Factors
- Personal Needs and Expectations of the Workforce.

Why is Wellbeing of the workforce in a school important?

- Wellbeing obviates negative functioning of individuals.

- Leaders who focus on wellbeing of their people tend to enjoy better relationships with them which in turn leads to high job-related wellbeing and job satisfaction for all.

- People who have a high sense of wellbeing and job satisfaction perform better. When people in our schools perform better, the result is that students' attainment and achievement improve, students' attendance increases, students behaviour improves and overall student outcomes improve.

- People who have a high sense of wellbeing and job satisfaction behave better. When people behave better, the place becomes a happy/great/wonderful place to work and becomes attractive to top talent.

- A school that has a high percentage of top talent performs better and whole school outcomes improve.

What is the level of Wellbeing in our school?

How well is our school?

Lack of wellbeing is strongly related to work stress

WHAT IS STRESS?

The definition is stress is elusive as it effects individuals in different ways. We know it includes mental health and is created through external and internal factors.

What are the possible causes of Stress in schools?

School leaders are required to not only meet performance objectives consistently for all within their team or school but to also attend to attract, retain, motivate staff. The pressure to deliver the best possible outcomes can cause them to place additional pressures consciously or unconsciously on the workforce which have far reaching negative effects including stress and the symptoms of stress in our schools.

Stress may arise from the following internal factors:

a. Increased emphasis on teachers' performance and accountability

b. Emotional demands made on teachers by students, parents, management.

c. Feeling undervalued

d. Inadequate pay

e. Poor working conditions

f. No involvement in decision making

g. Low control over time

h. Low collegial support

i. Lack of community between co-workers

j. Unfairness or disrespect

k. Loneliness

l. Poor student behaviour

m. Poor/ ineffective leadership and management

n. Internal politics

o. Ineffective communication

p. Excessive working time or workload.

q. Ineffective change management

r. Mismatch between workplace and personal values.

Stress may arise from the following external factors:

a. Changing demands from government/policy makers/stakeholders

b. Government initiatives

c. Crises e.g. health as in COVID 19 pandemic, Civil unrest as in ENDSARS, Wars, Famine etc.

What are the signs of Stress in schools?

• Staff burnout – exhaustion, cynicism, sense of inefficacy.

• Increase occurrence of illness.

• Increase occurrence of absence/ increases absenteeism.

• Increase level of disputes and disaffection.

• Increase level of complaints and grievances.

- Reports of stress/being stresses/ feeling stressed.

- Poor staff performance, Poor students' performance.

- Difficulty in attracting new staff.

- Low staff morale.

- Resistance to change.

- A blame culture.

WHAT CAN LEADERS DO?

There is an inverse relationship between leadership and management skills and staff stress.

As a leader your focus needs to be on promoting wellbeing amongst the workforce in your school through appropriate strategies and school wide consultation and decision making.

You need to answer the question "How can we as a school demonstrate a commitment to wellbeing alongside fostering effective systems to support the workforce on a broad level?"

A. Think holistically about wellbeing.

Many things affect the wellbeing, and a leader must be aware of them. Factors such as physical health, financial security, job security, career satisfaction, emotional health, relationships contribute to a person's feeling of wellbeing. School leaders should as themselves that they can do within the confines of their team and organisation to promote wellbeing.

For example, with financial security, think not only of amount paid but also about ensuring salaries are paid consistently/regularly.

With career satisfaction, autonomy, doing meaningful work, professional growth, and progress help.

With physical health institutionalizing regular health checks, water breaks, healthy meals, mental health awareness talks and inhouse psychologist can be considered.

B. Go to the basics and ensure excellent working conditions.

Workplace conditions refer to the working environment and all existing conditions affecting people in the workplace. If people really make an organisation function, how great are their working conditions? Poor working conditions can cause long term health problems including stress, depression, and anxiety.

10 points to Think About:

1. Think Physical Environment

- Is it conducive for working?

- Is it safe?

- Are the amenities in good condition?

- Is it noisy?

- Is there a staff room?

- Is there a creche for staff children?

- Is there a gym?

2. Think Structure

Ensure effective Organisational structure including clarity of roles, responsibilities, reporting lines, processes, procedures, and expectations.

3. Think Working Hours

In a meta-review analysis of 25 studies in Europe, United States and Australia, involving over half a million participants, those spending 55 hours plus working per week were at greater risk of strokes than those working a standard 35-to-40-hour week. (Kivimaki, 2015)

- Are they enabling and realistic?

- Can they be flexible? Can people work parttime?

- Is there time off?

- Are there breaks during the day?

- Is there structured leave?

- Can a person take an extended unpaid leave and sabbatical?

4. Think Pay

- Is your pay structure fair?

- Are your people being adequately compensated when compared to industry/location/income?

- Are people being paid at the right time, regularly?

• Are there incentives and rewards?

5. Think Talent and Performance Management

• What structure is in place for talent management? Are your people being coached, supported, encouraged?

• What is the purpose of performance management in your school? Development or punitive?

6. Think Change Management

• How is organizational change managed and communicated?

• Do you build in time for adequate reflection, planning, implementation of change initiatives?

7. Think Relationships

- Institutionalize processes to promote positive working to avoid conflict and deal with unacceptable behaviour.

8. Think Workload

- Is it appropriate?

- Does it promote work life balance?

9. Think Resources

- Are resources readily available?

10. Think Communication

- Is it effective?

C. Promote a culture that promotes wellbeing

1. Set a climate for belonging: a feeling amongst employees that they are part of a group gives them a hard sense of purpose and identity within their work. Involve your team in decision making.

2. Convey the right mood: Be mindful of signals we convey to people through our communication, attitude, choice of words, body language. All these affect the mood and mindset of individuals. It affects the mood and mindset of individuals. It affects whether they feel positive about then jobs and organisation.

3. Ensure effective communication and be accessible: Active listening skills enables leaders to empathise with employees. Knowing that you are being listened to and your needs are being considered helps people feel valued. Share ways you are working on your own wellbeing.

4. Signal the importance of wellbeing: Invest time in ensuring conversations about wellbeing are happening in the school consistently. Invite expects to take whole school workshops. Within teams, leaders should be asked to keep the conversation going. They should ask about the wellbeing of their teams and be supported and coached to identity and address issues.

5. Reduce uncertainty and increase certainty in your school: Honesty, clarity of expectations and priorities, autonomy and involvement in decision making help.

6. Help staff develop critical skill of energy management: Reduce rumination and circular thinking. Get more exercise, take work site breaks and work-related breaks, break down larger goals into smaller tasks.

"The higher your energy level, the more efficient your body. The more efficient your body, the better you feel, and the more you will use your talent to produce outstanding results."

- Anthony Robbins

7. Offer constructive feedback and praise: Positive reinforcement helps embed beneficial behaviors sand skills and leaders that adopt a strengths-based approach orient individuals towards both more productive behaviours and a healthier self-image.

Heaphy and Losada (2014) looked at 60 teams and concluded that the best performing ones averaged 5.6 compliments for every criticism. This contrasted significantly from the lowest performing teams, where there were 3 criticisms for every compliment. Positivity creates a healthier more progressive atmosphere.

8. Provide your people access to internal and external advice.

9. Maintain a pervasive focus on learning and development.

10. Gently but robustly address unhelpful attitudes: People will offer misinformed or stigmatizing beliefs about people who are struggling with their wellbeing or people who are making the best efforts to improve their wellbeing. Address this immediately.

D. Build systems that effectively monitor different aspects of school life/wellbeing through the year.

1. Observe: Keep an eye out for the signs of stress in your school. Keep records, check records, analyse data intentionally.

- Lateness

- Absenteeism

- Staff retention

- Staff recruitment

- Dip in performance

2. Ask: Go to source and ask them questions about their wellbeing. You can include a wellbeing check in as standard part of meetings. You may use a questionnaire, a focused group discussion or interviews. You may use a 3rd party to conduct the survey so people can feel confident responding honestly.

3. Act: The only thing worse than not asking for employee feedback is asking and not doing anything about it. Communicate what data reveals to your people and Act based on data. Include workforce wellbeing as KPI of team leaders. Include wellbeing as one of the values of your school. Create structures that support wellbeing at each level in the school and the school. Put in place coping strategies for both the individual and organisation.

E. You, the leader and your leadership style.

Wellbeing in the school, like all things starts with the quality of leadership in the team or school. Is the leader well? Do the leader's actions promote self wellbeing?

Leaders must walk the talk in a consistent manner. As a leader your actions have a consistent impact on the behavior of others. Be seen to be investing in your own well being.

No matter how much you say it is fine for your team to participate in health and wellness initiatives in your school, your body language and actions convey the most powerful message about what is encouraged and accepted.

If you never take breaks, if you work the latest every night, if you email/text at odd hours, if you never let your hair down, your people will feel the need to follow your lead.

As a leader you must demonstrate behaviour that are best for you and your team.

In a study done by Nielson et al, 2009, Transformational or Inspiring leadership was found to be associated with both job satisfaction and wellbeing.

Learning-centered leadership can help to promote wellbeing through laying emphasis on modelling. Modelling Is about the power of example but if leaders do not walk the talk in a consistent manner, then there is little probability of others of following.

Leaders should act as good role models to model improved behaviour including managing workload and work life balance showing you can achieve high performance with recovery time given.

WHAT ARE YOUR NEXT STEPS?

"Improving the health and well-being of our employees makes good business sense. As a leading provider of workplace health services, we see every day the difference it can make to a company's bottom line and the impact it can have on employee morale and motivation. It offers a "win-win" all round. Employees benefit from better support for their health. Companies benefit from less absence and improved productivity. And society benefits from improved public health."

- Steve Flanagan, Commercial Director, Bupa

"We are embedding health and well-being at the heart of our business strategy because our people are our greatest asset, and we recognize that a healthy, happy and committed workforce is vital to our business success."

- Alex Gourlay, MD, Boots UK

Further reading

https://www.hse.gov.uk/stress/standards/

https://www.verywellmind.com/how-to-deal-with-stress-at-work-3145273

https://www.mayoclinic.org/healthy-lifestyle/stress-management/in-depth/coping-with-stress/art20048369

https://www.health.harvard.edu/blog/how-to-handle-stress-at-work-2019041716436

About the Author

Dr. Abimbola Ogundere

Dr. Abimbola Ogundere is an Education advocate and Education leadership expert whose life's work is to create a generation of influential and impactful education leaders who identify and solve meaningful education problems at scale, all over the world.

She is a Medical doctor and Canadian certified Montessori teacher. She holds a master's degree in Public Health and a master's degree in Applied Educational Leadership and Management, both from the University of London, UK. She also holds a Women in Leadership certificate and a Certificate in School Management and Leadership from Harvard Business School, Boston, Massachusetts, United States.

She is the C.E.O of Kids' Court School, a renowned nursery and primary school in Lagos, Nigeria, founded in 2009.

Due to her enthusiasm for improving the quality of education received by the African child, in 2018, she founded Learning As I Teach Africa, an organisation dedicated to improving the quality of education received by the African child.

Learning As I Teach Africa, comprises of the **Learning As I Teach Foundation**, a non-for- profit organisation that seeks to bridge the access barrier to qualitative continuous professional development opportunities for the African teacher by providing opportunities such as **The Right Teacher Academy** for continuous professional development at minimal cost, and **Succeeding at Leading a Learning Community Coaching program** which empowers, equips and energizes school leaders to lead self and their schools to success and sustainability.

She is a thought leader and sought-after speaker on Education, Leadership and the Business of Education.

She is a published author of books including the bestselling The Right Teacher, The ABC of Teacher Professionalism, Hiring Right and The Complete Guide to Succeeding at School Leadership.

She is an Associate member of Women in Management, Business and Public Service (WIMBIZ) and a board member of The Dorcas Cancer Foundation, Melon Patch Farms and Schools Empowerment and support network SESN.

She is a career, life and relationship mentor for several young women and an avid supporter of women and children's rights and empowerment.

Dr. Abimbola Ogundere is married with three children.